I0704073

## DISCLAIMER AND TERMS OF USE AGREEMENT:

### (Please Read This Before Using This Report)

This information in this course is for educational and informational purposes only. The content is not presented by a professional, and therefore the information in this course should not be considered a substitute for professional advice. Always seek the advice of someone qualified in this field for any questions you may have.

The author and publisher of this course and the accompanying materials have used their best efforts in preparing this course. The author and publisher make no representation or warranties with respect to the accuracy, applicability, fitness, or completeness of the contents of this course. The information contained in this course is strictly for educational purposes. Therefore, if you wish to apply ideas contained in this course, you are taking full responsibility for your actions.

The author and publisher disclaim any warranties (express or implied), merchantability, or fitness for any particular purpose. The author and publisher shall in no event be held liable to any party for any direct, indirect, punitive, special, incidental or other consequential damages arising directly or indirectly from any use of this material, which is provided "as is", and without warranties.

As always, the advice of a competent legal, tax, accounting, medical or other professional should be sought. The author and publisher do not warrant the performance, effectiveness or applicability of any sites listed or linked to in this course.

All links are for information purposes only and are not warranted for content, accuracy or any other implied or explicit purpose.

# Contents

# Enthusiasm - The Best Weapon In The War Against Procrastination

Enthusiasm is what makes the difference between reaching our goals and giving up before we get started. Thomas Edison said, "If the only thing we leave our kids is the quality of enthusiasm, we will have given them an estate of incalculable value." Edison's research laboratory burned to the ground when he was 67. As the fire consumed his world-famous "invention factory," Edison told his children, "Kids, go get your mother. She'll never see another fire like this one." Edison knew that enthusiasm is the best antidote for tragedy, and it's the most powerful weapon to use in the war against procrastination.

I have learned that my level of enthusiasm has nothing to do with my feelings; my feelings wake up on a different side of the bed every day. To take control of my life, I must choose the way I feel-I can't let my feelings control me. Can you talk yourself into a positive frame of mind when you're discouraged? How do you keep yourself motivated? How do you stay focused when a job is tedious? How do you handle failure when your plan isn't going well?

- Stay away from negative people. Attitudes are contagious-negative people infect us with negative attitudes. Associate with positive thinkers; their self-confidence is contagious, too.

- Schedule difficult tasks for the time of day when your energy is highest. If you haven't determined the best time for you to tackle the day's least appealing jobs, try doing them as early as possible.

- Tackle a problem that's been a thorn in your side. When you get in the habit of making things happen, your enthusiasm goes through the roof. Inactivity is a major cause of depression and anxiety. (On the other hand, you can increase your energy level without eliminating other forces that cause procrastination; teenagers are particularly adept at expending enormous amounts of energy without getting anything done. Always remember that any technique is only effective when used as part of a total strategy.)

When you breeze through a task with particular ease and competence, make a note of the time of day. And ask yourself what other factors might have contributed to making you more

**How To Overcome Procrastination**

productive. When you start to discover a pattern, you will have found how to operate at a higher level every day. And when you identify the time of day when you are usually most efficient, schedule some of your least enjoyable tasks for that time.

We must continue to learn new things as if we were going to live forever, while living each day as if it were the last. Telling myself that "Today is the first day of the rest of my life" doesn't work for me. If today were the last day of my life, how would I live it? That is the question I ask myself when I must fight against the forces of procrastination.

Always remember that enthusiasm is a choice. Mark Twain said, "Do something every day that you don't want to do; this is the golden rule for acquiring the habit of doing your duty without pain."

# <u>How Conquering Procrastination Can Help You Reduce Stress</u>

I believe that procrastination is the No. 1 cause of stress in our society today. Throughout history, great thinkers have noted the connection between the failure to take action and the feeling of anxiety. The American philosopher William James once said, "Nothing is so fatiguing as the eternal hanging of an uncompleted task."

If you have the habit of putting off tasks you fear-if you tend to avoid situations and events that terrify you-your fears have grown out of proportion. Every time you decide not to do something because you're afraid of failing, your self-confidence takes another hit. There is only one way to overcome fear-you have to force yourself to do the thing you fear. When you face your fear and do it anyway, your confidence gets a big boost. Soon you will laugh at the imaginary fears that have kept you from becoming all that you can be. And you can do something about it today.

Establish goals. Prioritize. Measure your progress. Ask friends and office mates for feedback. Adjust your goals if necessary. Reward yourself when you finish jobs. If you're a leader, get procrastinators to encourage each other. Help them overcome their fear of getting things done. Find a mentor to help you overcome your fear. When I have to do the thing I fear, I recite a verse from the Bible: "I can do all things through Him who strengthens me." (Phil. 4:13)

Be as truthful as you can in your estimate of how long it will take to do the things you dislike. Many of the tasks we put off are simple ones. They cause an amount of stress in our lives that is altogether out of proportion to the time they require for completion. Think of when it took you much less time to do a dreaded job than you thought it would take. Can you learn something from that experience that could be applied to a task that has been left undone? Research shows that workers waste as much as a third of their workday. These same workers habitually complain about chronic stress caused by not having enough time to finish their jobs. Can you see the connection? The less you accomplish, the more you suffer from the sensation of stress and anxiety.

The only way to get at the root of the problem is by measuring how you spend your time. Keep a log of how much time you spend on things that you don't need to do. Make a note of the things

**How To Overcome Procrastination**

that could be done more efficiently. Try to do this for one full workday. When you analyze your list, you may be shocked at how much waste has seeped into your workday. Treat those items as a list of wasteful activities that need to be kept in check or completely eliminated. You probably don't control the cause of all the wasted time you've identified. Ask yourself what you can do to eliminate those things that you can control.

As the Mad Hatter said to Alice, "If you knew time as well as I do, you wouldn't talk about wasting it."

# How Planning Can Help You Conquer Procrastination

Benjamin Franklin, who knew how to conquer procrastination as well as anyone, said that "by failing to prepare you are preparing to fail." How do you plan your work? And if you don't plan, how do you know if you're reaching your goals? It's time to find out.

Make a list of everything you've been putting off at work. Not just the big things, but all the little things, too. Make another list of everything you've been putting off at home-large tasks and small ones. If you can't think of anything right away, walk around the house. Walk through the yard. It won't be hard to fill a page with projects that have been talked about, but not carried out.

Make another list of things you've neglected to do in the area of your personal relationships. That includes letters, emails, phone calls, visits, family trips, and vacations. Then make a list of all the things you've put off doing for yourself-a class you want to take, an exercise program you know you should start, or a bad habit you know you should eliminate.

Don't worry about priorities. Just get the juices flowing and write down everything that comes into your head. It may be hard to get started, but once you start the ideas will come more easily. Keep writing them down; you'll be amazed at how one thought triggers the next. Words will start to flow onto your paper or computer screen.

Now let me explain why I asked you to do this exercise. First, you've probably been putting off more things than you realized. That's the first step toward defeating procrastination-recognizing it as a problem. Procrastinators go to ridiculous extremes to explain their inability to take action. Accepting the truth that procrastination is a problem is the first step toward overcoming it.

Second, I hope this exercise has taught you the importance of getting started. The failure to take action breeds doubt, doubt gnaws at your self-confidence and your diminished self-confidence increases your indecision. The result is paralysis-and the vicious circle of inactivity keeps turning. After you recognize that procrastination is a problem, the next step is to focus on one thing you've been postponing. Take one thing you've been putting off and make something happen. You started your list with one thing; it led to another. Take one action and that action will trigger another.

**How To Overcome Procrastination**

Ask yourself how much time you waste in a day. Keep a log of how you spend your time. How do you plan your work to ensure that deadlines are met? Always ask yourself if the work needs to be done at all. According to research findings, we spend as much as 80% of our time on tasks that do not contribute to the success of our projects-many people load themselves down with work that is unnecessary, or that could be justifiably postponed. Learn what all successful people know: If you're failing to plan, you're planning to fail.

# How To Beat Procrastination - Stop Gathering Information!

Research shows that most of us spend up to 80% of our time on activities that have nothing to do with the success of our projects. We load ourselves down with endless tasks that keep us feeling busy, yet at the end of the day we wonder why we have accomplished so little.

Why do we miss deadlines, put off doing things we dislike, and accept stress and procrastination as a necessary part of life? What experiences have shaped the way you think about time? Do you need to rethink your views? If you were asked to speak to a group of students about the best way to use time, what would you say to them?

This quiz will help you identify areas where you can take action to overcome procrastination today:

- I often delay taking action and making decisions because I need to gather more facts.

- I have a hard time knowing when to wrap up the research phase of a project. I worry about not having enough information to complete it.

- I tend to get stuck in the middle of a project if changing circumstances suggest the need to make adjustments.

- I always feel that I'm using my time well as long as I'm gathering information for a project.

If you answered "yes" to any of the above statements, you need to recognize that procrastination is keeping you from achieving all that you can in life. Many people delay taking action by convincing themselves they need to gather more facts. Successful people know that effective decisions are based on opinions and experience first, facts second.

Set deadlines for yourself, even when you don't have to. You will never be able to gather all the facts. You must learn when to say enough. Make the best decision based on the facts you have now. The important thing is to act. We live in an increasingly complex world; our information-gathering techniques can't keep up with all the changing circumstances that affect our lives. We

## How To Overcome Procrastination

cannot control many of these circumstances, and we cannot control how other people respond to them.

Force yourself to act. Whatever decision we make today, we will have to rethink it-and almost certainly modify it-when circumstances change. No matter what you decide to do now, you will need to make corrections as you make progress toward your goal. Delaying a decision in order to gather more facts is one of the most common ways that people waste time.

Always ask yourself if a task needs to be done at all. The Bible says, "How forceful are right words! But what does your arguing prove?" Ask yourself: What do all my tasks prove? Focus on getting things done, rather than on filling your day with more activities than you can possibly get around to. If you want to overcome procrastination, stop gathering facts and get started on your project.

# How To Overcome Procrastination - Accept Responsibility

All procrastination is the result of deluding ourselves. Procrastinators deny reality, refusing to accept responsibility for their lives. To defeat procrastination, we must stop playing games with ourselves. You can't overcome procrastination until you accept the fact that you are responsible for what you make of your life. That may be more honesty than many people are capable of, but there is no other way to achieve a richer life.

The first step toward overcoming procrastination is recognizing that it's a problem. Procrastinators have big problems and small problems, but most of their problems are caused by procrastination.

**All procrastinators share certain traits:**

- They know what they should do about a problem, and in many cases they know what specific action needs to be taken. Yet they find reasons to avoid action.

- They are reluctant to do anything about a problem now, but vow to take action at some vague time in the future.

- They promise to take action when the "right" circumstances present themselves. By making performance of the job depend on something else, they justify their decision to delay action. They delude themselves into thinking that their hands are tied. They would like to do something but can't-it's not their fault.

Research shows that you can develop new habits in just two weeks if you're serious about changing. Think about people you know who always get things done. What are their work habits? How do they approach unappealing tasks? How do they stay focused?

**Here are some simple tips that can help you take charge of your life today:**

- Mentally prepare yourself to be productive. I begin every day in prayer and meditation. I keep inspirational messages where I can see them. Then I visualize my success during the day.

**How To Overcome Procrastination**

Procrastination is a real monster, and it won't go away unless we do something about it every day. If I'm passionate about a job, I can get it done at any time of day and under any circumstances-the problem is when to tackle the hardest and most tedious jobs. Always ask: At what time of day am I most productive? Most people say they're most productive early in the morning; by mid-afternoon it's harder for them to sit still and concentrate on work. Try to schedule the hard jobs for your most productive time.

- Don't over-socialize at work. Office chitchat and gossip keep many people from getting more accomplished. Let people know when you don't want to be disturbed. Think about the things in your work environment that contribute to staying focused. What things distract you or make you want to postpone a job? How can you redesign your environment to eliminate causes of procrastination? (A workspace doesn't have to be neat, if you know where to find things.)

We are not victims of our circumstances. You can overcome procrastination now-you can do the things that need to be done. And you can learn to distinguish between the things that need to be done now and the things that can wait.

# How To Overcome Procrastination - It All Depends On You

Procrastinators put off all the hard jobs. But they get stuck in a vicious circle of postponing the easy jobs, too. And the longer they put them off, the harder the jobs are when they finally get around to them. Successful people fight the same war against procrastination that we all face, but they have learned not to give in. They know that procrastination is the cause of many of the problems we face in our daily lives.

Procrastination creates a never-ending cycle of frustration, stress, and defeat. When people learn how to take charge of their lives, their self-esteem improves and their confidence grows. No matter how long you've been struggling with the demon of procrastination, you can start to take control of your life today by tackling a job or responsibility you've been putting off.

There are many books, online courses, and methods for changing your life and developing your personal and professional skills. I believe that procrastination is the root cause of the majority of problems that people face. Best-selling author Wayne Dyer said: "Procrastination is one of the most common and deadliest of diseases, and its toll on success and happiness is heavy."

Take the first step toward a richer life by getting serious about overcoming procrastination. The following quiz will help you identify areas where you can take action today.

1. I have written a list of my life-time goals.

2. I have written a list of my short-term goals (6 months or less).

3. I keep these lists where I can see them; they help me stay focused.

4. I establish priorities; some things that seem urgent are not important when I focus on the big picture. Yes ( ) No ( )
5. Once I've made a decision, I don't worry about whether I made the right decision or not-I just concentrate on getting the job done.

6. I know when to say "no" to avoid taking on too many jobs at once.

## How To Overcome Procrastination

7. I live in the present; I focus on what I'm doing now instead of dwelling on what I should have done in the past.

8. When I've done the best I can, I know when to wind up a job-spending more time on the same job only keeps me from starting something new.

If you answered "no" to any of the above statements, make a commitment to take corrective action today. Choose one item and do something about it. Don't move on to the next item until you can truthfully answer "yes" to the previous one. You've taken the first step by reading this far; now take the next step and do something you've been putting off. If you want to change, you can-the best time is now.

# How To Overcome Procrastination - Just Do It!

The first step toward overcoming procrastination is recognizing that procrastination is a problem. Procrastinators have big problems and small problems, but the fact is that most of their problems are caused by procrastination.

**All procrastinators share certain traits:**

- Procrastinators know what they should do about a problem, and in many cases they know what specific action needs to be taken. Yet they find reasons to avoid action.

- Procrastinators are reluctant to do anything about a problem now, vowing to take action at some vague time in the future.

- Procrastinators promise to take action when the "right" circumstances present themselves. By making performance of the job depend on something else, they justify their decision to delay action. They delude themselves into thinking that their hands are tied. They would like to do something but can't-it's not their fault.

- All procrastination is the result of deluding ourselves. Procrastinators deny reality, refusing to accept responsibility for their lives. To defeat procrastination, we must stop playing games with ourselves. You can't overcome procrastination until you accept the fact that you are responsible for what you make of your life. That may be more honesty than many people are capable of, but there is no other way to achieve a fulfilling life.

We are not victims of our circumstances. You can do the things that need to be done. And you can learn to distinguish between the things that need to be done now and the things that can wait.

1. Have you written a list of your life's goals?

2. Have you have written a list of short-term goals (3-6 months)?

**How To Overcome Procrastination**

3. Do you keep these lists where you can see them?

4. Do you set clear priorities? Do some things that seem urgent take on less importance when you focus on your larger goals?

5. Do you know when to say "no" to keep from burdening yourself with more jobs than you can finish?

6. Do you live in the present? Do you focus on what you're doing now, rather than on the things you should have done in the past?

7. When you've given your best effort, do you know when to wrap up a project?-Do you feel that spending more time on it will only keep you from starting your next project?

Did you answer "no" to any of the above questions? If you did, you need to make a commitment to do something about it today. Choose an item and make up your mind that you're going to do something about it. Don't worry about the next item until you've made a dent in the first one. Now that you've taken the first step by reading this article, take the next step and finish a job you've been postponing-there will never be a better time than now.

# How To Take Charge Of Your Life - No More Procrastination

To be successful in the battle against procrastination, you must establish priorities and stick to them. Successful people have learned that they must do the hard jobs whether they're in the mood or not.

Take this quiz to find out if you need to get more serious about procrastination:

- Do you set priorities?

- Do you get the hard jobs done whether you're in the mood or not?

- Do you spend most of your time working on tasks that you need to finish this week?

- Do you spend time each day working on your long-term goals?

- Do you have a system for measuring your progress?

- Do you have a filing system for each of your long-range projects?

If you answered "no" to any of the above questions, you need to get more serious about procrastination. Ask yourself if you're happy living with the consequences of procrastination. Do you have justifiable reasons for postponing tasks, or have you simply developed the habit of putting things off?

**- Establish your priorities.** If you don't make a list of your priorities every day, why don't you? And if you do make a list, ask yourself how you rank items in order of importance.

**- Force yourself to act**. Set deadlines for yourself, even when you don't have to. You need to spend most of your time on this week's projects, but try to spend a little time every day on long-term goals.

## How To Overcome Procrastination

**- Spend 75% of your time on the things you need to finish this week.** Dedicate the rest of your time to projects that need to be finished in the next six months. If you don't have a list of deadlines for the next six months, make one now. What have you done so far on each of these projects? How are you measuring your progress on each one?

**- Keep a file for each long-range project.** This can be a folder with the deadline date in big letters on the outside. Write down target milestones for each big project. (A milestone is a deadline for finishing one part of a project.)

Wasting time on tasks that don't contribute to the success of our projects is one of the most insidious forms of procrastination. When you decide to rush into something on the spur of the moment, always ask yourself if it's the best way to spend your time. Could I accomplish more with the time I have by doing a different task? Which of these two tasks will make a greater contribution to getting the job done?

Don't put yourself in the position of Shakespeare's King Richard II, who was forced to say: "I wasted time, and now time doth wasted me." Get serious about procrastination today.

# Overcome Procrastination And Start Living A Richer Life Today

- Do you make excuses when you miss deadlines?
- Do you tend to look for excuses to explain why you didn't do something, rather than take action to finish the job?
- Is there a good reason why you didn't finish the job?
- How important is finishing the job?
- Have you written down a plan for finishing it as soon as possible?

Stop blaming failures on the circumstances around you. The next time you hear yourself making excuses, it may help to remember what the American poet Henry Wadsworth Longfellow said about the predicaments procrastinators get themselves into: "It takes less time to do a thing right than explain why you did it wrong."

Do you see yourself as a victim of events and circumstances? Do you complain more than other people? What do you do when you procrastinate? How do you spend your time when you've decided not to do something you should do? Are you serious about wanting to change? Are there hidden causes of your procrastination that you need to discover?

Procrastinators are always able to find reasons for not getting started. To take control of your life, you have to accept responsibility for everything that happens with your projects. When you fail, analyze what happened and ask yourself if you could have produced a better outcome by doing something differently. This will improve your ability to successfully complete the next project, and you'll be ready to take the first step to get started on it. Identify what needs to be done and do it now-circumstances will never be perfect for starting the job.

The only way to break out of the vicious circle of procrastination is by asking hard questions. We are not victims of our circumstances. You can do the things that need to be done. And you can learn to distinguish between the things that need to be done now and the things that can wait. Whenever you consider delaying a project, ask yourself the following questions:

- What are the benefits of waiting?

**How To Overcome Procrastination**

- Do I have a justifiable reason for postponing this project?
- Do I want to go on living with the consequences of leaving things undone?

Look in the mirror and ask yourself if you're delaying a task for a justifiable reason. Put all your reasons for wanting to delay the project under a microscope; consider the possibility that your reasons are merely excuses for not getting started. Think about the last time you delayed a project. What benefits did you expect to receive by waiting? Write them down. Now ask yourself how the project came out. Did the project benefit from the delay?

Justifiable reasons-or if you're just making excuses. What would have happened if you had pushed forward on the project anyway? And always remind yourself of what Napoleon Hill said about waiting: "Do not wait. The time will never be just right."

# The Best Cure For Procrastination - Your Vision

Have you discovered your purpose in life? Do you have long-term goals? Finding and focusing on your long-term goals is a powerful cure for procrastination. A vision is simply a statement of what you want to achieve in life, and how you plan to achieve it. Without a vision, it's easy to fall into a lifestyle of procrastination. And without a clear statement of your vision, you're more likely to give up on projects in the face of difficulties.

If you haven't written your vision, you need to make this your No. 1 priority. Your goals and your attention will shift from one project to the next, year after year, if you don't have a vision to guide you.

**- Make a written list of your lifetime goals.** Wishing won't make it happen-writing down a goal is the first action you can take to conquer procrastination. One research study discovered that people who write down their goals earn ten times more than people who don't. You may think you have a goal, but if you haven't written it down, research suggests your chances of accomplishing it are small.

**- Break down your long-term goals into measurable tasks.** This is the only way you can stay focused enough to keep moving toward your long-term goals. Without a series of clearly-defined milestones to measure your progress, you can delude yourself into thinking that you're moving toward a goal when in fact you haven't taken the first step yet. Do you constantly miss deadlines? Do you make up reasons to justify why you didn't finish an important task, rather than tackling it and getting it done? Are you sincere enough to recognize the real reason why you missed your deadline? Do you have a written plan of attack for finishing the job without further delay?

**- Perfectionism is one of the main causes of procrastination.** Recognize the difference between striving for excellence and getting stuck in a vicious circle of perfectionism. Ask yourself what type of work demands perfectionism. If the job you're doing is not the type that requires perfectionism, then remember that your goal must be excellence rather than perfection.

## How To Overcome Procrastination

**- Always keep a journal or idea book with you.** Use spare time to jot down ideas about how you plan to attack your next goal. When you're working on one project, what do you do when you get random ideas about other things? Do you write them down? Writing is a great way to use spare time and unleash your creative thinking and problem-solving skills. Don't worry about spelling or grammar-just get your thoughts down as quickly as you can. If you need to show what you've written to someone else, you can revise it later.

Remind yourself that every task you face today is part of a divine plan for your life. "There is a divinity that shapes our ends, rough-hew them how we will," Shakespeare wrote. You were created to accomplish more than you think you can-do some "rough hewing" on your life's goals today.

# There's Only One Way To Defeat Procrastination - Do Something!

Are you a habitual procrastinator? This quiz will help you identify areas where you can take action to overcome procrastination today:

- Do you have a filing system for keeping track of your long-term and short-term projects?

- Do you believe that the right atmosphere plays an important role in determining your productivity? Do you try to design work areas so that they help you to stay focused on the task you're doing now?

- Do you congratulate yourself when you complete a job on time?

- Do you eliminate unnecessary tasks from your daily schedule?

- Are you usually accurate in deciding which jobs can be delayed for a justifiable reason?

- Do you stay focused on your strengths, rather than constantly worrying about your weaknesses?

Don't deceive yourself-procrastination is the main reason people fail to live fulfilling and prosperous lives. How do you usually keep yourself moving forward when you would rather put something off? If you answered "no" to any of the above questions, make a commitment to do something about it. The following tips can help you defeat the procrastination monster today:

- Keep a diary of your successes. When you force yourself to move forward to make something happen, write it down. Make a note of how it felt to complete the job successfully. The next time you can't get started on a hard task, or when you want to give up, open your diary a read about one of your past successes. This can energize you and keep you moving forward.

**How To Overcome Procrastination**

- When you have difficult assignments, make them team projects if you can. Delegate or outsource the things you dislike or don't do well. Concentrate on your strengths. Don't let your weaknesses paralyze you.

- When you complete a hard job, reward yourself. Do you give yourself a reward when you stick with a difficult job and see it through to the end? What things bring you joy? How can you use these things as rewards for jobs completed? Sometimes the best reward is time for rest and recuperation. As Albert Einstein said, "The idle man does not know what it is to enjoy rest."

- Use your time well. One clear symptom of procrastination is the habit of filling your day with unnecessary work, or work that can be justifiably delayed. Create the right atmosphere at work for staying focused on your priorities. As the English statesman and author Lord Chesterfield said, "The less one has to do, the less time one finds to do it." Make a list of what you most regret not doing in your life because of the poor decisions you made about how to use your time. There's only one way to defeat procrastination-Do something about it now.

# Tips For Overcoming Procrastination - Raise Your Expectations

Many people believe they cannot change. "I yam what I yam," the cartoon character Popeye habitually explains. Before any change can happen in your life, you have to believe that a transformation is possible. There comes a time when we must say: "I am willing to change."

Beware of mental locks. In A Whack on the Side of the Head, Roger von Oech offers a list of what he calls "mental locks." To break free of a life of procrastination and mediocrity, we must guard our minds against thoughts that destroy our expectations of success. This quiz will help you identify areas where you can take concrete action to change your attitude. Answer "yes" if you have ever thought or said the following:

- I've never been a creative person.
- Stay where you are until you have perfect visibility.
- Follow the rules.
- Please be logical!
- That doesn't sound like the right answer.
- Please be practical about this!
- Avoid making mistakes at all costs.
- If this doesn't work, I'll look like a fool.
- That's out of my area of expertise.

Choose one of your "yes" items and reflect on the last time you said or thought it. Did thinking or saying it cause you to procrastinate or give up? Our thoughts and words influence the outcome of our efforts-what you say is what you get.

Even a simple quiz like the one you just took can be a great opportunity to improve your ability to make things happen and get things done. Don't expect to change your attitude by rushing through all the points at once. Work on one thing every day until people ask you what happened. When others start to see a change in your attitude, you'll know that you're winning the war against procrastination.

**How To Overcome Procrastination**

It starts in your mind. When you have a total determination to get things done, you tap into unused capabilities you never knew you had-abilities most human beings never use. When you expect to be successful, you jump at the opportunity to do the very things that used to cause you to procrastinate.

Never lose your sense of humor. The great nineteenth-century Scottish physicist, James Clerk Maxwell, was told by his superiors at Cambridge University that he would be expected to attend a compulsory church service at 6:00 a.m. "Aye," Maxwell said, "I suppose I could stay up that late."

Always remember to beware of the mental locks that threaten to keep us in a vicious circle of procrastination and defeat. Make up your mind to rise above the level of mediocrity-give yourself a whack on the side of the head and do it.

# Tips For Students Who Want To Overcome Procrastination

Take this quiz to find out if you-or any students in your family-need to get serious about overcoming procrastination:

- Do you put off assignments until the last possible hour because you like to think of yourself as the type of person who works best under pressure?

- Do you write down your priorities before you start projects? Do many things seem unimportant when you look at them in the light of these priorities?

- Do you ask yourself which of several tasks is the most important one before you rush into an assignment?

- Do you concentrate on finishing an assignment when you're in danger of missing a deadline, rather than complaining that you never have enough time to get your work done?

- Do you make sure your friends know when not to disturb you?

- Do you turn off the TV and your phone when you need to work on an important assignment? Do you concentrate completely on what you're doing now, rather than dwelling on what you did in the past?

- When you've done the best you can, are you content to wrap up a project and hand it in as it is?-Do you generally make good estimates of how much time it will take to finish an assignment?

If you answered "no" to any of the above questions but the first one (I hope you answered "no" to that one), you can develop better study habits by getting serious about procrastination. Try doing the hardest assignments first. Sandwich a difficult assignment between two of your favorite ones.

## How To Overcome Procrastination

Most students dread writing assignments, putting them off to the last possible minute. Writing is one of the most important skills a student can develop. Here are some tips from great writers that can help you conquer the procrastination monster:

- Winston Churchill wrote about 5 million words in his lifetime. That's the equivalent of ten thousand 500-word articles, so he must have enjoyed writing very much. And he wrote well-well enough to win a Nobel Prize for literature. Churchill once said: "When you're going through Hell, keep going." To paraphrase that advice for all students struggling with a writing assignment: When you don't know what to write, keep writing.

- Don't be a bleeder. (Journalists who agonize over every word they write are known in their profession as "bleeders.") The faster you write, the more you'll enjoy writing. Jack London, one of my favorite writers when I was a student, said that "you can't wait for inspiration; you have to go after it with a club."

- Another Nobel Prize Laureate, John Steinbeck, said: "Write freely and as rapidly as possible and throw the whole thing on paper. Never correct or rewrite until the whole thing is down. Rewrite in process is usually found to be an excuse for not going on." In other words, rewriting before you finish a first draft is an excuse for procrastination.

# <u>Tired Of Putting Things Off? - Put An End To Procrastination Today</u>

I've been planning to write a novel for the last twenty years. I keep putting it off. Best-selling author John Grisham wrote his first novel while working full-time as an attorney; he was as busy as the rest of us, but he found a way to accomplish his dream. How did he do it? He beat procrastination by forcing himself to get up earlier every morning so he could work on his book before he went to work.

Take this quiz to find out if you need to put an end to procrastination:

- Do you write down your priorities? Do some things seem less urgent when you look at them in the light of your priorities?

- Do you ask yourself which of several tasks is the most important one before you decide what task to tackle next?
- Do you accept full responsibility for missing a deadline, rather than blaming it on forces beyond your control?

- Do you focus on finishing a job on time, rather than looking for excuses to explain why you're going to miss another deadline?

- Do you make sure people know when not to disturb you?

- Do you have a habit of turning off the phone when you need to concentrate completely on a job? Do you focus on the job at hand, rather than fretting over what went wrong in the past?

- When you've done your best, do you know when to wrap up a project?-Do you feel that spending more time on it will only keep you from starting your next job?

If you answered "yes" to all of the above questions, congratulations-you're in John Grisham's league. If you answered "no" to any of the above questions, pick one and make a commitment to do something about it today. Ask yourself if you have really considered all the consequences

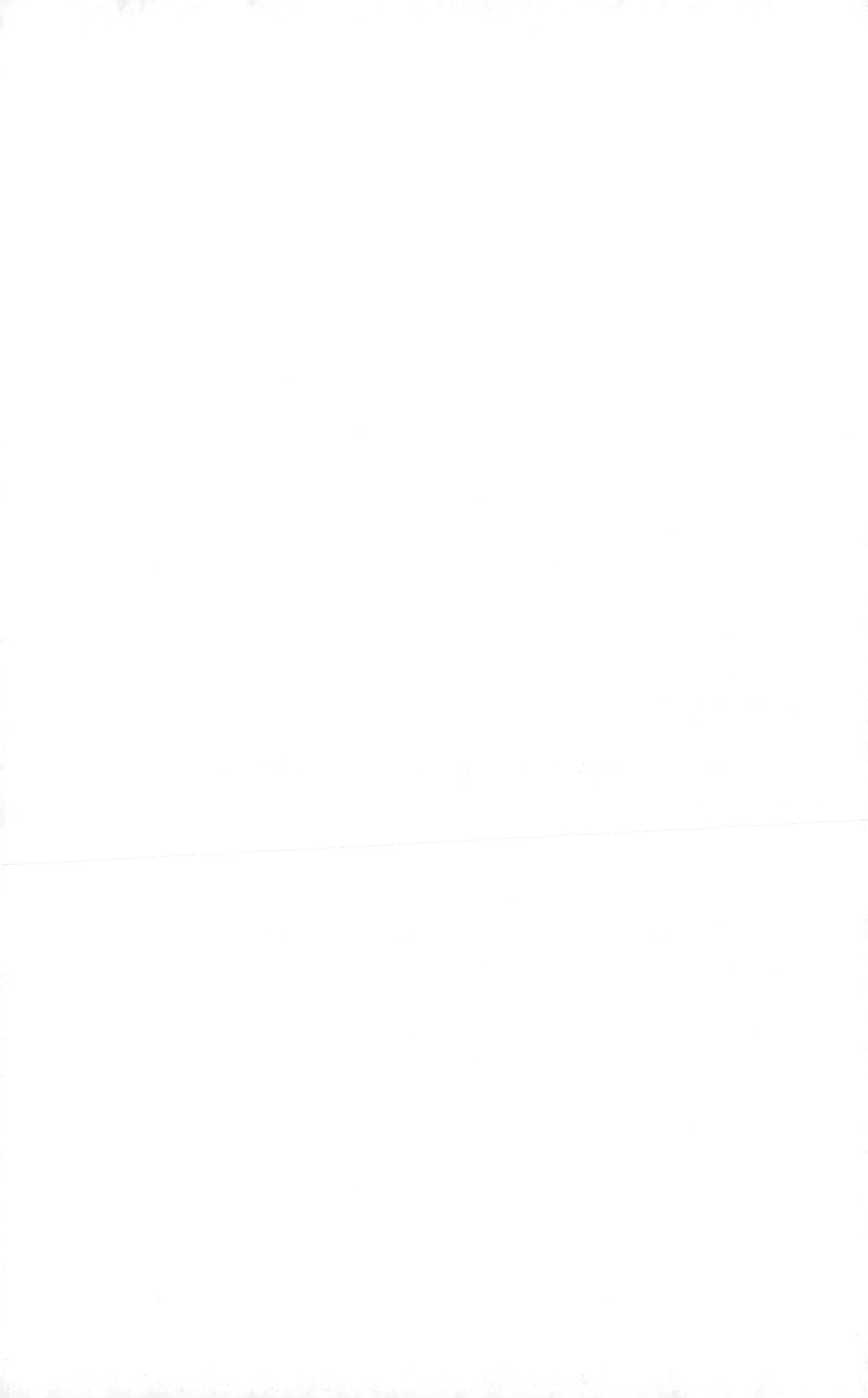

## How To Overcome Procrastination

of procrastination. Do you want to live with them forever? Do you have a legitimate reason for postponing jobs? And after thinking about these questions, ask yourself if you delay tasks for justifiable reasons-or if you just make excuses to procrastinate. Here's what I've learned to do:

- Always remind yourself that you have as much time as people who do great things.

- Make your best estimate of how much time a task will take.

- Write an inspirational phrase on a 3 x 5 card and use it whenever the procrastination monster pops up.

Shakespeare said, "Thoughts are but dreams till their effects be tried." You've taken the first step to defeat procrastination by reading this article; now take the next step and tackle a job you know you should have started a long time ago. I took my next step this morning-I got up earlier than usual to start my novel.

# Win The War Against Procrastination - The Battle Begins In Your Mind

Mark Twain had something to say about almost any topic you can imagine. On the subject of how to avoid procrastination, Twain said, "Never put off until tomorrow what you can do the day after tomorrow." Everyone can enjoy the humor in Twain's comment. But for many of us, Twain's insight on the danger of procrastination is painfully true.

You can take the first step toward a more satisfying life by getting serious about overcoming procrastination. And the place to get started is in your own mind-that's where the war is won or lost. To overcome procrastination, you have to change your attitude. All successful people know that you have a better chance of completing a job when you approach it with a positive attitude:

- Your attitude is a choice. Many people procrastinate because they tell themselves that they will increase their chances of success if they wait for all the circumstances to be "right" before tackling a project. To be successful, you must force yourself to make a decision and do something no matter what the circumstances say.

- Your attitude determines the outcome of your actions. People who are successful at what they do are rarely those with the greatest natural ability or the highest IQ. People who are constantly able to complete jobs successfully have a positive attitude-they believe they can complete the job.

- You cannot control the past, so move on. Thinking about how you might have responded differently to a difficult problem in the past is an important part of preparing to be a better problem-solver today. Analyze what you could have done differently, chalk it up to experience, and then forget about it.

The following quiz will help you identify areas where you can take action today. Answer "yes" to each statement that describes you.

1. I don't wait for the "right" set of circumstances to tackle a job-I know the circumstances will never be perfect.

**How To Overcome Procrastination**

2. I believe my project will be successful if I give it my best effort.

3. When I fail, I don't blame circumstances beyond my control; I ask myself what I could have done differently to bring about a different result.

4. I don't fret over decisions once I've made them-I stay focused on what I'm doing in the present.

5. I know when to wrap up a job-if I spend more time on it I'm only making up excuses for not starting something new.

If you answered "no" to any of the above statements, make a commitment to change your attitude today. Choose one item and do something about it. Don't move on to the next item until you can truthfully answer "yes" to the previous one. "Be not the slave of your own past," Ralph Waldo Emerson said. Cut the chains of procrastination and start living life to the fullest.

# Don't Let Procrastination Keep You Down

Author Denis Waitley believes that one of the main causes of procrastination is a fear of success. "People procrastinate because they are afraid of the success that they know will result if they move ahead now," he explains. And Miguel Cervantes, the author of Don Quijote, wrote that "delay always breeds danger, and to protract a great design is often to ruin it."

Great thinkers throughout history have known that procrastination is the main reason people fail to live more rewarding and more prosperous lives. Take this quiz to find out if a fear of success is causing procrastination in your life:

- Are you passionate about the life you're living? Have you discovered your mission in life? Do you have a written list of long-term and short-term goals you want to achieve?

- Do you always ask yourself which of several tasks is the best way to spend your time? Do you always ask which task should be your higher priority in view of your short-term and long-term goals?

- If you won a large amount of money, would you continuing living as you are now? Are you living the kind of life that even money can't buy?

- Do you concentrate on the job you're doing in the present, rather than feeling sorry for yourself because you aren't living the life you wish you were living?

If you answered "yes" to all of the above questions, you're winning the war against procrastination. If you answered "no" to any of the questions, you need to recognize the possibility that procrastination is keeping you from living a richer life.

Ask yourself why you haven't written a vision for your life. What are the benefits of establishing priorities? Do you postpone tasks for justifiable reasons, or do you simply look for excuses to procrastinate.

**How To Overcome Procrastination**

Always ask yourself if a job needs to be done at all. Make a list of what you most regret not having done in your life because of the poor decisions you made in the past about how to spend your time. According to research findings, we spend as much as 80% of our time on tasks that do not contribute to the success of our projects. Many people load themselves down with work that is unnecessary or that could be justifiably postponed.

Are you passionate about your life and work? Ask yourself how you would spend your time if you won ten million dollars and never had to work again. These questions can lead to some surprising revelations about what your priorities should be. You may discover that you would be happier by making a career change, although in most cases people don't need to switch careers to start living a richer life-they just need to know what they really want.

As the novelist George Eliot said, "It's never too late to be the person you could have been." Today is a good day to start.

# How A Positive Attitude Can Help You Overcome Procrastination

The following quiz will help you identify areas where a negative attitude has been keeping you from taking charge of your life. Answer "yes" to the statements that describe you.

1. I get discouraged when I think about all the problems I have.

2. I often wonder why my life is not as rewarding as it could be; many people around me seem to be living more satisfying lives than I am.

3. I have trouble focusing on my goals; I'm easily distracted at work.

4. I tend to put off getting started on projects because I'm always thinking about the things that can go wrong.

If you answered "yes" to any of the above statements, make a commitment to start retooling your attitude today. Read motivational books, listen to inspirational recordings, and associate with positive thinkers.

We cause our own feelings; I am the major cause of my own problems. Don't let a negative attitude stand in the way of your happiness in life. Never make an important decision when you're feeling down. What is your best time for making decisions? What is your worst time? What is your best time for working on difficult tasks? Is there a time of day when you tend to procrastinate more? Is there a time of day when you tend to procrastinate less?

Here are some tips for improving your attitude that can help you take the first steps toward overcoming the procrastination monster:

- Focus on the result you want to achieve. The more you focus on problems, the more discouraged you're likely to get. If you're not getting what you want out of life, you probably suffer from a lack of focus. This is why procrastination is such a dangerous demon-it prevents

**How To Overcome Procrastination**

us from focusing on our goals. Procrastinators focus on all the reasons not to move forward, instead of focusing on the goal they want to achieve.

- Give your full attention to whatever you're doing. When you concentrate on the things that can go wrong, you can't stay focused on the job you're doing. Failure is the inevitable consequence of a lack of focus; if I think I'm going to do a bad job, I probably will-or I may never get started at all.

- Don't focus on all the things that can go wrong. Focusing on the hazards involved in trying to do something will almost always convince you to give up before you start.

I'm not advising you to throw caution to the wind. Every task we undertake has things that can go wrong. Simply said, it's enough to know what the dangers are, be prepared to respond to them, and then move ahead with the project-confident in your ability to handle whatever comes up. People who dwell on all the things that can go wrong never get anything done. Productive people have learned to focus on opportunities-concentrate on the benefits of successfully completing a project and you will have won a major battle in the war against procrastination.

# How To Beat Procrastination - Face Your Fear And Do It Anyway

Many people procrastinate because they fear they'll look foolish if they fail. It took Edison more than 10,000 failed attempts to discover the tungsten filament that worked in the incandescent light bulb. A reporter asked him how he managed to go on working in the face of so many failures. Edison told the reporter that each failure gave him hope; every time he failed, he knew he was one step closer to finding the answer. Edison believed that "many of life's failures are people who did not realize how close they were to success when they gave up."

Successful people make more mistakes than others because they never stop trying to achieve new goals. If you're not making mistakes, you probably aren't attempting enough. Force yourself to get out of your comfort zone and take action.

One kind of fear is good: You should feel guilty when you don't finish a job, and you should fear the consequences of sub-par performance. That kind of fear can be a powerful motivator to perform at your highest level.

Does it help you to think about the consequences of procrastination? Knowing the consequences of our actions doesn't always keep us from doing the wrong thing, of course. If the consequences of not finishing an important job are not getting you motivated to start it, why not? What's going on? You have to start asking these questions to get at the roots of the problem. What is really causing you to procrastinate?

English actor Christopher Parker said, "Procrastination is like a credit card: It's a lot of fun until you get the bill." We have all heard smokers say, "I want to stop smoking but I can't"-as they light another cigarette. The person who says this doesn't know what his real problem is. As we watch them smoke, it's clear that they don't want to quit smoking at all.

Talking about quitting lets smokers go on enjoying their habit while deluding themselves into thinking that they really are making an effort to stop. They want to avoid the part of smoking that causes them to get lung cancer-we have no reason to doubt that. But it's plain to see that they enjoy all the other perks they get from smoking. Smokers are not likely to give up their habit until they are able to face the real cause of their problem.

Think of a time when you could have procrastinated but didn't. How did you feel? How could you turn that into a good habit? When fear threatens to immobilize you, ask yourself this question: What's the worst thing that can happen? Write down your answer as precisely as you can. Be prepared to accept the worst. Now write down as many solutions as you can think of. Decide on the best action and do it. Ralph Waldo Emerson said, "Don't waste your life in doubts and fears: spend yourself on the work before you, well assured that the right performance of this hour's duties will be the best preparation for the hours and ages that follow it." Face your fear and do it anyway.

# How To Defeat Procrastination And Get The Most Out Of Life

I believe that procrastination keeps the majority of human beings from getting the most out of life. What is it exactly? The word procrastination literally means to leave something "for tomorrow." It comes from the Latin words pro (for) and cras (tomorrow). Procrastination is the postponement of something that you know you should do.

There are no "born" procrastinators; they develop their bad habits one step at a time. And that's how you can develop new habits to defeat procrastination-one step at a time. But you have to take the first step. You will never become a more active, take-charge person by reading articles and books on how to overcome procrastination. The best advice in the world will do you no good at all unless you act on it.

So I encourage you to make a commitment to act on the tips you find here. You may not agree with everything I say; I fight a daily battle against procrastination, too, and I don't always win. But you and I are on the same side-procrastination is our common enemy, and we both want to beat it.

Procrastination keeps people from living their best lives. Why do we procrastinate? There are many reasons: indecision, stress, fatigue, depression, a desire to gather information, disorganization, fear of failure, and even fear of success. You can't defeat procrastination overnight-if you're a procrastinator, you have been accumulating bad habits over a lifetime. But you can defeat procrastination by making a disciplined effort to get at the roots of the problem.

- Tip No. 1: Take full responsibility for your failures. One of the main causes of procrastination is the habit many people have of blaming their failures on circumstances. When you tell yourself that failures are caused by circumstances beyond your control, you are preparing yourself for a lifetime of procrastination.

- Tip No. 2: Just do it. Successful people know that their success depends on a commitment to do whatever it takes to reach a goal. Success in all projects, large and small, is determined by the actions you take and your ability to stay focused on your goals. This is true whether your goal is to reduce clutter at home, lose weight, restore a relationship, or complete a major project

**How To Overcome Procrastination**

at work. Projects come in all different shapes, sizes, and levels of importance, but the principles that determine their success or failure are always the same: focus, determination, self-discipline, and confidence.

- Tip No. 3: Establish your priorities. What does it mean to change? To change is to choose a behavior different from the one you're using now. We all have to fight the drift toward procrastination every day. If you're losing the war against procrastination, you need to get your priorities right. Make a list of your priorities at work and in your relationships.

Make a commitment to make something happen in at least one of your high-priority items every day. The novelist George Eliot said, "It's never too late to be the person you could have been." The best time to start is now.

## How To Defeat Procrastination - Believe You Can

The power of belief is a key to success in everything we do. Whether your goal is to rise to the top of your profession or to be a better weekend golfer, you have a better chance of success if you believe you'll be successful. And by believing that you can defeat procrastination, you can start to take charge of your life today.

Learn how to control your negative thoughts. When your mind says you can't do something, refuse to listen to it. Don't express your negative thoughts in words; tell your mind-and say it out loud-that you're going to do what it takes to get the job done.

It isn't easy, but it's worth the effort. Many people procrastinate because they've made up their minds that they're going to fail. If you are one of these people, the most important thing you can do today is to stop believing what the procrastination demon has been telling you.

Human beings are unique because of our ability to change-to become more than what we are. But before we can change, we must be able to accept full responsibility for everything we do. Smokers who say they "hate" smoking are deluding themselves-as an ex-smoker, I claim some authority on this topic.

We have a choice. People smoke because they want to smoke. It may be very hard for many people to quit smoking, but that's not the point-they'll never quit as long as they lie to themselves about the real cause of their habit. People are able to quit smoking when they really want to quit.

Take this quiz to find out if negative thoughts are causing procrastination in your life:

- When you tackle a job, do you expect to be successful? Do you think you'll be able to complete the job successfully by giving it your best effort?

- Do you visualize your success? When you face a difficult task and feel like giving up, are you able to give yourself a pep talk to stay motivated?

**How To Overcome Procrastination**

- When friends, family members, or others help you recognize a habit that you need to change, are you able to recognize the truth in what they say? Do you believe you can change your bad habits?

- Do you accept responsibility when your projects fail, rather than looking for something beyond your control to blame it on?

- When your mind says you're going to fail, do you try to replace these negative thoughts with positive ones?

If you answered "no" to any of the above questions, ask yourself what you can do to approach life with a more positive attitude. Do you want to go on living with negative thoughts, doubts, and fears? Are there any benefits of clinging to a negative attitude?

We can change bad habits by wanting to change them. And you can defeat the habit of procrastination in your life-especially if you believe you can.

# How To Overcome Procrastination - Set Daily Goals

The surest way to know that you can do something is to have done it before. When you set daily goals for yourself, you develop the habit of getting things done. When the procrastination demon appears, you know how to force yourself to push ahead because you've done it before. If you feel like you're losing the battle against procrastination, one of the most effective strategies for taking charge of your life is to get in the habit of accomplishing daily goals.

Set a goal every day, and achieve it. It's easy to get discouraged when your projects don't seem to be going anywhere. We all need a long-term vision to guide our day-to-day efforts, but many people with high goals develop a negative attitude when they think they're not making progress. That's why it's important to set achievable goals every day. The more goals you achieve, the more positive your attitude will be.

Set weekly and monthly goals. Your short-term goals are milestones that keep you moving toward long-term goals. They help you know if you're going in the right direction. When a long-term goal seems far away, it's easy to feel discouraged. Breaking down a large project into smaller segments makes it easier to stay focused. Congratulate yourself when you achieve daily and weekly goals, and give yourself a special reward when you achieve a monthly goal.

It's important to experience the satisfaction and rewards of successfully completing jobs. When you force yourself to keep moving until you finish a project, it's easier to get started on the next one. Don't be surprised if you feel yourself grappling with the drift toward procrastination now and then-it may never go away completely. All successful people learn how to identify the procrastination monster, and they know what to do about it when it threatens:

- Successful people use their time well. When an urgent task threatens to pull them away from what they're doing, they don't rush into it just because it seems urgent. They always ask: Which of these two things is higher on my list of priorities?

- They turn off the phone from time to time. Can you get more done by leaving a voice message and turning the phone off during certain periods of the day? The telephone is one of the most

**How To Overcome Procrastination**

insidious thieves of our time. It's urgent but rarely important. It shoves out the less urgent but more important things.

- They keep a log of how they use their time. If they miss a deadline, they plan how to finish the remainder of their work and estimate as accurately as possible when it will be done.

- They develop a routine. They set an objective to accomplish every morning and every afternoon.

- They leave time in their daily schedule for contingencies.

- They always think twice before postponing a task. Successful people know that pushing themselves to accomplish daily goals makes them more likely to achieve long-term goals.

# Increasing Your Energy Can Help You Defeat Procrastination

Lack of exercise is a well-known cause of chronic fatigue. Research studies have found that of all people who visit doctors to complain about problems of fatigue, only about 20% require medical treatment. What about the other 80%? They suffer from the effects of a sedentary lifestyle-in the overwhelming majority of cases the cause of chronic fatigue is a lack of exercise. And people who complain of chronic fatigue also tend to be victims of procrastination.

When is your energy highest? Why do you think that is? Do you stay depressed for long periods? What foods give you energy? What foods slow you down? What foods and beverages help you sleep better? What foods and beverages rob you of sleep?

- Boost your energy. You're more likely to tackle the jobs you've been putting off when you feel energized. The best way to increase your energy level is by exercising regularly. More energy in your life will make the tedious jobs less tedious because you become better at getting them done. The more energy you have, the faster you get them done and the better you feel about yourself.

- Monitor your habits and lifestyle. I am working on this article at a stand-up desk. Winston Churchill, Ernest Hemingway, and Thomas Wolfe are just a few of the writers who discovered that they worked faster and better while standing. Thomas Jefferson drafted the Declaration of Independence on a stand-up desk that he designed for himself. A stand-up desk keeps my posture right-and it keeps me focused on my work without squirming around as I tend to do when I'm seated for extended periods of time. A high stool lets me alternate between sitting and standing. I'm amazed at how my productivity and concentration have increased since I started to use a stand-up desk.

- Be grateful you have the opportunity to do the hard jobs. I think about the woman who finished a regulation 26.2-mile marathon at the age of 92. It's easier to do things you normally dread when you're conscious of your blessings; be grateful you have the opportunity to do the hard jobs. When you see things in their proper perspective, your time is too precious to be squandered in a life of procrastination.

**How To Overcome Procrastination**

- Research shows that certain foods contribute to deep sleep. I have always been a sound sleeper. Here are some of my favorite late-night foods: bananas, peanut butter, whole wheat bread, and potatoes. I also know what foods and beverages keep me tossing and turning at night; when I indulge in them after dark I pay the price the next day-my energy is low. Pay attention to what works for you.

Following a regular exercise program, eating the right foods, alternating between sitting and standing, and doing some simple stretching during the day-all of these techniques keep my energy high. And when I feel energized, I'm less likely to fall into the procrastination game. As the American humorist Will Rogers said, "Even if you're on the right track, you'll get run over if you just sit there."

# No More Excuses - How To Overcome Procrastination Today

People get stuck in a lifestyle of procrastination because they believe their own excuses for not taking action. Procrastination is the main reason that people fail to live richer and more fulfilling lives. If you're stuck in a rut of continual procrastination, make up your mind to stop making excuses.

If you've been making excuses for putting things off, here's how to take charge of your life. First, think about all the things you've been postponing-at work, at home, in your personal relationships, or for your personal development. Make a list.

Now choose one thing on that list that you can do something about today. Write down every excuse you've given yourself for not having done anything about it yet. Ask yourself if you have considered all the consequences of your procrastination in this area. Do you want to live with them? Do you have a legitimate reason for postponing this job?

You have to be honest about this or it won't work. Forget about what other people think; look in the mirror and ask the hard questions. If you have a legitimate reason for delaying action in this area, move on to another item on the list. Find something that you can make happen today, simply by deciding to make it happen. Now do it. When you've completed this task successfully, your satisfaction will motivate you to repeat this process with another item on your list.

Successful people know that their accomplishments depend on two things: taking action and staying focused on their goals. People who are successful in any business or profession have an ability to make things happen. All successful people win the war against procrastination because they develop certain traits. To defeat procrastination and get all you want out of life, you must:

- Know what you want.
- Force yourself to take action.
- Be willing to make mistakes and learn from them.
- Stop making excuses!

**How To Overcome Procrastination**

Now go back to your list and choose another project. Write down every excuse you've been giving yourself for not getting started, or for leaving it unfinished. Put as many things on the list as you can think of. Now try to eliminate one excuse at a time. Ask yourself hard questions: Why do I have to postpone this project? Is it necessary to go on postponing it? If Bill Gates were in my situation, would he postpone it? What will happen if I keep putting this off? If I keep putting this off, when will I get it done? Can I get started on it now? What part of the job could I complete now? If I postpone this job now, what other job will I tackle to make better use of my time?

As you eliminate your excuses, think of what you can do today to make this project happen, and do it. Anne Frank wrote in her diary, "How wonderful it is that nobody need wait a single moment before starting to improve the world." Make a decision to start improving your world today.

# Time - Your Most Valuable Asset In The War Against Procrastination

Research shows that people spend most of their time and effort working on activities that have nothing to do with the success of their projects. I'm convinced that procrastination is the main reason people fail to live richer lives. If you want to get serious about eliminating the habit of procrastination, you can start right now by recognizing that your most valuable asset is time.

- Learn how to use your time efficiently. Make sure that people know when you don't want to be interrupted-don't blame other people when you don't have enough time to finish a task. When you miss a deadline, plan how you're going to finish the remainder of the work instead of making excuses about why you didn't get it done on time. Then do it.

- Procrastination is the No. 1 cause of stress. Do you ever wonder why the most successful entrepreneurs-people like Bill Gates, for instance-always seem so relaxed in interviews and public appearances? They work harder than most of us and they make billion-dollar decisions that the rest of us will never have to face in life, yet they never seem stressed out, worried, or depressed. Why not? Research shows that stress is caused by leaving too many things undone. That's why habitual procrastinators always complain about chronic fatigue-putting things off creates enormous stress in our lives, which manifests itself as fatigue.

- Break down your long-term goals into manageable segments and milestones. Without a way of measuring your progress on long-term goals, you can easily delude yourself into believing that you're making progress when you're just spinning your wheels. Setting project milestones is a good way to measure your progress and stay focused.

- Reserve some time each day for working on your long-term projects. Spend most of your time on the things that need to be done this week, but try to spend some time each day on work that helps you make progress toward your long-term goals. The tasks that help you achieve long-term goals are easy to leave undone. They don't seem urgent in the way that telephone calls seem urgent, but they usually represent our most important goals in life. In many cases, these larger goals get pushed off the radar screen by the countless distractions and "urgent" but unimportant things that demand our attention throughout the day.

**How To Overcome Procrastination**

You need to spend 75 to 80% of your time on jobs you have to wrap up this week. Dedicate the rest of your time to projects that need to be finished in the next six months. Have you set milestones for these projects? How are you measuring your progress on each project?

Always ask yourself: What have I learned about the consequences of procrastination, based on the decisions I made-or failed to make-yesterday? Never lose sight of what's most important in life, and ask yourself every day: If I only get one thing done today, what must that one thing be? Then get it done.

# Why You Need An Action Plan To Defeat Procrastination

Procrastination is the main reason people fail to live richer lives. If you haven't been reaching your goals, you may need to make a greater commitment. And the only reliable measure of commitment is action. When you delay getting started on a job or fail to complete a job you've already started, always ask yourself why you're not working on it:

1. I can't do it and I don't want to do it.
2. I can do it but I don't want to.
3. I want to do it but I can't.
4. I can do it and I want to.

If you're honest with yourself, you can probably get started on the fourth type of projects today. If you do, you will have taken the first step toward defeating the monster of procrastination.

Research shows that you can develop new habits in just two weeks if you are serious about changing. Taking action and staying focused on your goals is what makes private dreams and corporate missions come true. The tasks people avoid are almost always the ones on which the success of their projects depends. Make a list of your least favorite tasks. Ask yourself how you approach them. Do you tackle them first or leave them for last?

Think about people you know who always get things done. What are their work habits? How do they approach unappealing jobs? How do they stay focused? Try doing the least enjoyable jobs first, or put a task you dislike between your favorite ones. As Mark Twain said, "If you have to swallow a frog, don't stare at it too long."

If you have trouble making commitments because you think you won't be able to live up to them, you may want to try the method that served Thomas Edison so well. When Edison had an idea, he would go public by announcing his invention at a press conference. Having told the world about it, he went into his laboratory and invented it.

You may not want to try this out at work any time soon, but I'm sure you can think of many ways to apply the technique of "going public" in other areas of your life. The point is: Thomas Edison,

**How To Overcome Procrastination**

the greatest and most productive inventor in the history of the United States, understood how important it is to keep from drifting into inactivity. His technique for defeating procrastination was an extraordinary one, and he used it to achieve extraordinary results.

Put your favorite inspirational sayings where you can see them. Let people know when you don't want to be disturbed. Think about the things in your environment that help you get into the flow of your work. What things distract you or make you want to postpone a job? How can you design or rearrange your environment to eliminate causes of procrastination?

Thomas Edison said, "If we did all the things we were capable of doing, we would literally astound ourselves." Do something today that you've been putting off and start astounding yourself.

This Product Is Brought To You By

# DAVID A OSEI